MAKE YOUR

HARD LOTION

A HEALING ALTERNATIVE TO TRADITIONAL LOTIONS

Amberlee Rynn & Caleb Warnock

THE BACKYARD RENAISSANCE COLLECTION

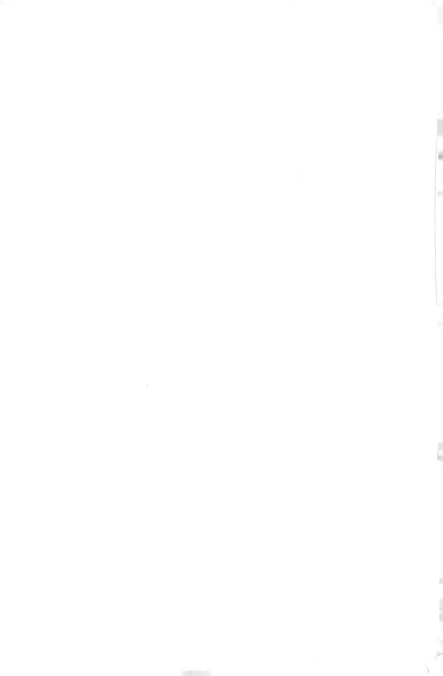

DISCOVER THE LONG-LOST SKILLS OF SELF-RELIANCE

My name is Caleb Warnock, and I've been working for years to learn how to return to forgotten skills, the skills of our ancestors. As our world becomes increasingly unstable, self-reliance becomes invaluable. Throughout this series, *The Backyard Renaissance*, I will share with you the lost skills of self-sufficiency and healthy living. Come with me and other do-it-yourself experimenters, and rediscover the joys and success of simple self-reliance.

FAMILIUS

Published by Familius LLC, www.familius.com

Familius books are available at special discounts for bulk purchases for sales promotions, family or corporate use. Special editions, including personalized covers, excerpts of existing books, or books with corporate logos, can be created in large quantities for special needs. For more information, contact Premium Sales at 559-876-2170 or email specialmarkets@familius.com.

Library of Congress Catalog-in-Publication Data
2015931054   pISBN 978-1-939629-73-9   eISBN 978-1-942672-06-7

Cover and book design by David Miles
Edited by Sarah Echard

10 9 8 7 6 5 4 3 2 1

First Edition

CONTENTS

THE STORY OF AMBERLEE'S HARD LOTION BARS 7

OILS FOR HEALTHY SKIN 12

NATURAL SEED BUTTERS FOR SOFT SKIN 18

BEESWAX TO SEAL IT ALL IN 20

ESSENTIAL OILS FOR FRAGRANCE 22

MAKING HARD LOTION 23

BASIC RECIPES 26

RECIPE VARIATIONS 34

STARTING A LOTION BAR BUSINESS 37

FREQUENTLY ASKED QUESTIONS 44

DEFINITIONS 50

SUPPLY SOURCES 52

Heated lotion bar ingredients can scald skin and cause permanent injury. Do not use hot ingredients near children. Do not use hot ingredients if they cannot be handled safely. The authors are not responsible or liable for any injury that may result from following the instructions in this book.

THE STORY OF AMBERLEE'S HARD LOTION BARS

Store-bought lotion can contain over twenty different ingredients, many with mysterious-sounding names and acronyms. Most health-conscious people read the labels on their food, but when was the last time you read the list of ingredients on the back of your bottle of lotion?

The lotion I personally used before I began making my own lotion had twenty-one ingredients, and I began to wonder what these ingredients were. A little research led me to the Environmental Working Group (EWG), a nationwide environmental health research and advocacy organization. According to EWG's research, twelve of the ingredients in my favorite lotion had toxicity concerns—and I was putting them all over my body! As a chemist, I work with toxic chemicals, and I am required, for my own safety, to wear gloves and goggles and work under a ventilated hood to protect me from the chemicals' toxic effects. Then I go home and practically bathe in lotion containing preservative chemicals that produce formaldehyde. Not so smart. Lotion is designed to be absorbed into the skin, so guess where all those chemicals are going?

I began looking at the Campaign for Safe Cosmetics website (www.safecosmetics.org) to find healthier alternatives. I could buy a safe lotion in a six-ounce tube for $10, but that was a huge price jump from the $6 for twenty ounces that I had been paying for my previous lotion. I learned that I could make my own lotion for much cheaper, but I was troubled to learn that homemade lotion required patience with blending, blending, and more blending—and if I didn't want to add a chemical emulsifier, I'd have to keep the lotion in the fridge. I do not enjoy smearing myself with frigid lotion.

I felt defeated, so I kept buying lotion that I was sure was going to poison me.

One day, while I was standing in the grocery aisle, staring at my unhappy prospects, my husband picked up a little tin of Burt's Bees Miracle Salve®. He wanted it to try on his very cracked and split knuckles. We purchased it, and within weeks, the salve had improved my husband's knuckles more than any lotion had ever done. Curious, I tried it on my skin, and it lived up to its name: "miracle." The ingredient list was made up of different oils and beeswax. This got me thinking about the possibility of creating a different kind of lotion, one that did not require any water. I wondered if it could it work.

THE PROBLEM WITH LIQUID LOTION

Lotion is a combination of water, oil, and other compounds that are either natural or man-made. These ingredients are blended to create a substance that moisturizes the skin by increasing hydration and softness. Moisturizers often include a combination of oils, emollients (any substance which softens or soothes the skin), and humectants (any substance that pulls moisture from the air into the skin).

Most of the toxic chemicals in store-bought lotion are added to give the lotion fragrance, to keep the water and the oil mixed together, and to keep the mixture from spoiling. Water supports life of all kinds, including bacteria. When water is added into lotion, it creates a place for bacteria to thrive and multiply. Because of this risk, store-bought lotion contains added chemicals to kill any bacteria that may grow.

Whether your lotion is store-bought or homemade, if your lotion has water in the ingredients, it will need an emulsifier.

It is simple science: water and oil do not mix. An emulsifier is a substance that holds water and oil together. Water and oil can be mixed together for a very short period of time without an emulsifier, but eventually the two will separate. Without an emulsifier, lotion must to be kept in a refrigerator to slow that separation. In addition, homemade lotion that does not contain chemicals to kill bacterial growth has a shelf life of about two weeks—maybe a month if it is kept refrigerated—even with an emulsifier added.

How do we fix all these problems with lotion? We stop making lotion with water.

Without water in the lotion recipe, it is no longer necessary to include an emulsifying agent. Without water, the lotion is inhospitable to bacteria. And without water, the blending required to make liquid lotion is no longer necessary. Making hard lotion bars instead of liquid lotion solves the need for chemical additives.

Best of all, hard lotion bars are simple and cost effective. A hard lotion bar, which is also sometimes called a massage bar, can be made with as few as three ingredients. The basic formula for hard lotion is oil, butter, and wax.

HOW TO USE HARD LOTION: RUB BAR AGAINST SKIN WHEREVER LOTION IS DESIRED. THE NATURAL WARMTH OF YOUR BODY WILL MELT A THIN LAYER FROM THE HARD LOTION BAR. ONE OR TWO PASSES WITH THE BAR IS ENOUGH. THEN MASSAGE THIS LAYER OF LOTION INTO YOUR SKIN.

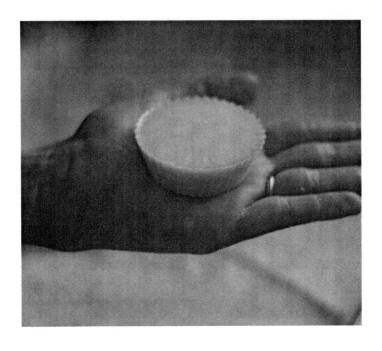

OiLS fOR HEALTHY SKiN

The kinds of natural oils you choose to use when creating your lotion bars make a big difference. The three oils I use for my own lotion bars are coconut oil, avocado oil, and either apricot kernel oil or apricot seed oil. Each of these oils has different properties, and you can use them to customize the hard lotion bar to meet your skin's needs.

COCONUT OIL

The oil pressed from coconuts comes from the inner white flesh of the coconut and is a good everyday moisturizer. The properties of coconut oil meet a broad spectrum of your skin's needs. It has a natural SPF of 5, so it protects skin from the sun's harmful UV rays. It is also a humectant, so it pulls moisture from the air. It can even be used to strengthen hair. However, coconut oil can have a drying effect on some people's skin. Another downside is that coconut oil is slightly "comedogenic," meaning that it can clog pores.

Some skin really loves coconut oil; some skin doesn't. Experiment with it. If it doesn't work for your skin, you can use the rest in cooking applications, as long as it is high-quality oil.

AVOCADO OIL

This oil comes from the green flesh of the avocado and is my personal favorite. Avocado oil is high in vitamin E, which promotes healing for your skin. It has high skin penetration and a fast absorption rate. It also promotes nutrient absorption through the skin. However, avocado oil can leave a waxy feeling on the skin for some people. Again, experiment to see what your skin likes.

APRICOT KERNEL OIL

This oil comes from the apricot kernel and is a good choice for those who experience the greasy residue that can be left by oils. Apricot kernel oil has a very similar lipid content to skin, which allows for complete absorption and leaves behind minimal residue. It is good for softening and soothing skin. Apricot kernal oil is also recommended to help combat the effects of aging on skin.

TIP: I CHOOSE TO USE COCONUT, AVOCADO, AND APRI-
COT KERNEL OILS BECAUSE THEY MEET A WIDE VARI-
ETY OF NEEDS AND THEY ARE COST EFFECTIVE. THESE
ARE VERY EASY TO FIND AT YOUR LOCAL HEALTH FOOD
STORE AND ARE REASONABLY PRICED. THERE ARE
DOZENS OF DIFFERENT OILS THAT CAN BE USED IN
HARD LOTION BARS, BUT THEY QUICKLY BECOME EX-
PENSIVE. SOME OF THE MORE EXPENSIVE AND DIFFI-
CULT-TO-FIND OILS INCLUDE TAMANU OIL, WHICH HAS
TREMENDOUS SKIN HEALING PROPERTIES, AND PRIM-
ROSE OIL, WHICH IS GOOD FOR DIMINISHING SCARS
AND REDUCING WRINKLES.

COLD-PRESSED AND EXPELLER-PRESSED OILS

Be sure to get cold-pressed oils. Cold pressing is a method
of extracting oil from seeds and nuts without using any heat.
Heat can change the chemical composition of oil or make the
oil go rancid. Heat can also damage the oil through a process
called oxidizing, which creates free radicals that can damage
the cells in your body. You do not want to put things containing
free radicals on your skin, as those free radicals can be ab-

sorbed into the body. Cold-pressed oil avoids these problems.

An expeller press is used to remove oil from crushed seeds or nuts by pressure. Expeller pressing can be a method of cold pressing, depending on how the manufacturer treats the process. It is possible for mechanical-expeller presses to get quite hot. According to Fooducate.com, in the United States, there is no legal definition of what is required for an oil to be considered "cold-pressed."[1] In Europe, cold-pressed oils must not be exposed to temperatures above 90 degrees Fahrenheit, which is difficult to attain when using a mechanical press. So even cold-pressed oils made in the United States may have been exposed to high heat. Exposing oils to heat in the pressing process helps get far more oil out of the seeds and nuts.

Using a chemical solvent is the cheapest and most efficient way to remove the most oil from seeds and nuts. Hexane is the chemical mostly widely used for this purpose, but hexane is poisonous. Hexane is a chemical made from crude oil, a colorless liquid with a slightly disagreeable odor, according to the Agency for Toxic Substances and Disease Registry. Hexane is known to negatively affect the human nervous and reproductive systems. There is no information about how hexane might affect human health in low exposure over the long term and no information about hexane exposure in children. In laboratory studies, animals exposed to high levels of hexane in the air had signs of nerve damage. Some animals also had lung damage. In other studies, rats exposed to very high levels of hexane showed damage to sperm-forming cells.[2]

The only way to know for sure whether an oil is genuinely cold pressed and not exposed to temperatures above 90 degrees or to chemicals like hexane is to do research about individual oil manufacturers.

A NOTE ABOUT OLIVE OIL: OLIVE OIL CAN BE USED TO MAKE HARD LOTION BARS, BUT FINDING GOOD-QUALITY AND UNADULTERATED OIL CAN BE CHALLENGING AND EXPENSIVE. AS A GENERAL RULE, CHEAP OLIVE OIL IS PROBABLY NOT PURE OR COLD-PRESSED. ACCORDING TO A JANUARY 2014 *NEW YORK TIMES* EDITORIAL CALLED "EXTRA VIRGIN SUICIDE," BY NICHOLAS BLECHMAN, A 2010 STUDY BY RESEARCHERS AT THE UNIVERSITY OF CALIFORNIA, DAVIS, FOUND THAT 69 PERCENT OF IMPORTED OLIVE OIL LABELED "EXTRA VIRGIN" DID NOT MEET THE STANDARDS FOR THAT LABEL. SOME OIL PRODUCERS WAIT WEEKS OR EVEN MONTHS TO PROCESS THE OLIVES. OTHER PRODUCERS MIX OLIVE OIL WITH SOYBEAN OIL OR OTHER CHEAP OILS, AND SOME MIX CHEAP OILS WITH BETA CAROTENE AND CHLOROPHYLL TO PRODUCE FAKE OLIVE

AS WITH THE OILS, LOOK FOR COLD-PRESSED BUT-
S. COCOA BUTTER AND SHEA BUTTER ARE VERY
MON, BUT MANGO BUTTER MAY BE A LITTLE MORE
FICULT TO FIND FROM A LOCAL STORE. ALL ARE
DILY AVAILABLE ONLINE.

OIL. IN ADDITION, OIL MAY BE LEGALLY LABELED
"IMPORTED FROM ITALY" AS LONG AS THE OIL LEFT
FROM AN ITALIAN DOCK, BUT MOST OFTEN THESE OILS
ARE MADE FROM OLIVES GROWN, PROCESSED, AND
PRESSED IN SPAIN, MOROCCO, AND TUNISIA.[3] FOR ALL
OF THESE REASONS, I DO NOT USE OLIVE OIL TO MAKE
LOTION BARS.

EESWAX TO SEAL IT ALL IN

eeswax forms a protective layer over skin so all
that moisture stays locked in and skin can heal.
Beeswax will form a waterproof barrier to keep
your hands from drying out. You may even notice
re reapplying less lotion after washing your hands.
g on how processed the beeswax you choose is, it
n its antimicrobial properties. Beeswax is also lightly
tive, with a natural SPF of 5. If you process your own
it is antimicrobial; if it doesn't smell like honey, it has
its antimicrobial properties because it has been so
d filtered.

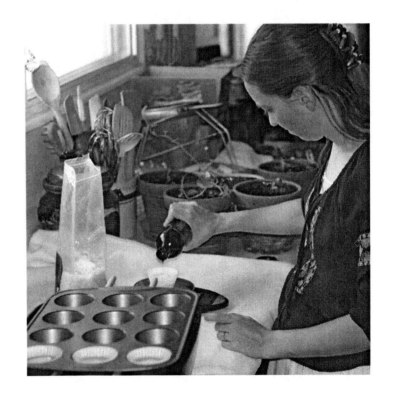

NATURAL SEED BUTTERS FOR SOFT SKIN

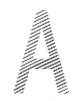butter made from a plant is a puree of the meat of the seed or the seed itself. For example, coconut butter is simply coconut meat blended until it is creamy.*

*AN EXCEPTION TO THIS DEFINITION IS MANGO BUT-TER, WHICH IS ACTUALLY MANGO KERNEL OIL, BUT BE-CAUSE IT IS SOLID AND CREAMY AT ROOM TEMPERA-TURE, IT IS LABELED A BUTTER. IN THIS CASE, THE WORD "BUTTER" IS USED AS A DESCRIPTION OF THE TEXTURE OF THE OIL.

Adding a butter to the hard lotion bar makes it feel very creamy on skin. Butter made from plants also adds some healing properties to the hard lotion. The ones I use personal-ly are cocoa butter, which is made from the whole cocoa bean; shea butter, which is made from a nut; and mango butter.

COCOA BUTT

Cocoa butter comes from making ch beans. It smells just like chocolate and is day, whole-body moisturizing; it is an er and soothes your skin; it is pretty solid so it helps keep the hard lotion more soli tures; and it is a humectant, so it pulls m

SHEA BUTT

Shea butter comes from the African she slight odor, depending on the quality. I temperature. Shea butter has a thick cc tense moisturizer for problem areas— luses and dry skin. If you use it on your little heavy, almost like Vaseline®. It is mectant, so if very dry skin is a problem

MANGO BU

Mango butter comes from the mango at room temperature. Mango butter is properties to cocoa butter, so it is goo turizing.

TI
TE
CO
DI
RE

B

that you
Depend
may reta
UV prote
beeswax
not kept
heated a

OIL. IN ADDITION, OIL MAY BE LEGALLY LABELED "IMPORTED FROM ITALY" AS LONG AS THE OIL LEFT FROM AN ITALIAN DOCK, BUT MOST OFTEN THESE OILS ARE MADE FROM OLIVES GROWN, PROCESSED, AND PRESSED IN SPAIN, MOROCCO, AND TUNISIA.[3] FOR ALL OF THESE REASONS, I DO NOT USE OLIVE OIL TO MAKE LOTION BARS.

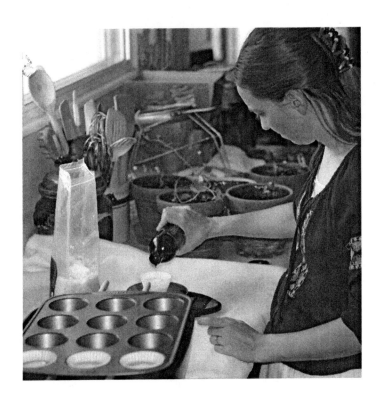

NATURAL SEED BUTTERS FOR SOFT SKIN

A butter made from a plant is a puree of the meat of the seed or the seed itself. For example, coconut butter is simply coconut meat blended until it is creamy.*

*AN EXCEPTION TO THIS DEFINITION IS MANGO BUTTER, WHICH IS ACTUALLY MANGO KERNEL OIL, BUT BECAUSE IT IS SOLID AND CREAMY AT ROOM TEMPERATURE, IT IS LABELED A BUTTER. IN THIS CASE, THE WORD "BUTTER" IS USED AS A DESCRIPTION OF THE TEXTURE OF THE OIL.

Adding a butter to the hard lotion bar makes it feel very creamy on skin. Butter made from plants also adds some healing properties to the hard lotion. The ones I use personally are cocoa butter, which is made from the whole cocoa bean; shea butter, which is made from a nut; and mango butter.

COCOA BUTTER

Cocoa butter comes from making chocolate from cocoa beans. It smells just like chocolate and is really good for everyday, whole-body moisturizing; it is an emollient, so it softens and soothes your skin; it is pretty solid at room temperature, so it helps keep the hard lotion more solid in warmer temperatures; and it is a humectant, so it pulls moisture from the air.

SHEA BUTTER

Shea butter comes from the African shea nut and may have a slight odor, depending on the quality. It is a soft solid at room temperature. Shea butter has a thick consistency and is an intense moisturizer for problem areas—perfect for healing calluses and dry skin. If you use it on your entire body, it can be a little heavy, almost like Vaseline®. It is an emollient and a humectant, so if very dry skin is a problem, shea butter will help.

MANGO BUTTER

Mango butter comes from the mango seed and is a soft solid at room temperature. Mango butter is odorless but has similar properties to cocoa butter, so it is good for whole-body moisturizing.

BEESWAX TO SEAL IT ALL IN

Beeswax forms a protective layer over skin so all that moisture stays locked in and skin can heal. Beeswax will form a waterproof barrier to keep your hands from drying out. You may even notice that you're reapplying less lotion after washing your hands. Depending on how processed the beeswax you choose is, it may retain its antimicrobial properties. Beeswax is also lightly UV protective, with a natural SPF of 5. If you process your own beeswax, it is antimicrobial; if it doesn't smell like honey, it has not kept its antimicrobial properties because it has been so heated and filtered.

TIP: CARNAUBA WAX CAN BE SUBSTITUTED FOR BEES-
WAX IF YOU ARE VEGAN. CARNAUBA COMES FROM A
TREE.

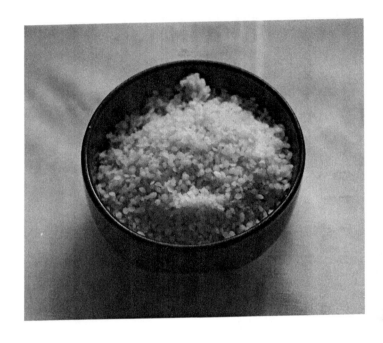

ESSENTIAL OILS FOR FRAGRANCE

The hard lotion bars I sell contain essential oils to make them scented, but I don't put essential oils in my personal bars because I don't want the bars to be scented. When I want the medicinal properties of the essential oils, I put them directly on my skin after I've applied my hard lotion.

Any essential oil can be used in hard lotion. I add essential oils after the other ingredients are already melted because the long exposure to heat can break the oils down. I add three to five drops of oil per ounce of hard lotion. Three drops are sufficient for stronger scents like lavender or peppermint, whereas five drops or more of citrus oils may be necessary.

TIP: CITRUS OILS CAN BE PHOTOSENSITIZING, MEANING THEY MAY MAKE YOUR SKIN MORE SENSITIVE TO SUNLIGHT AND BURN EASIER, SO AVOID SUNLIGHT OR UV RAYS FOR TWENTY-FOUR HOURS AFTER APPLICATION.

MAKING HARD LOTION

Now that you know what oil, butter, and wax you prefer, you can start making your hard lotion. Bar production is another area in which you can customize the product to your skin and climate. Some people will make two types of bars, a summer bar and a winter bar. Summer bars have more beeswax in them so that the lotion bar does not melt as easily in ambient heat, and winter bars have less beeswax so that they melt more easily. My recipe seems to hold up well in both summer and winter use, so I make the same recipe for both seasons.

TOOLS YOU WILL NEED

- **1 metal muffin pan.** This must be metal, not silicone, because you will be carrying and moving this pan with hot oils in it.
- **Set of 12 silicone muffin cup liners.** A set costs about $10 on Amazon.com or at a craft store. Only silicone muffin cup liners should be used so that you can cleanly and

easily get the hardened lotion bars out of the pan when they are done. The metal muffin pan alone will not work.

- **1 electric skillet OR double boiler.** I use an electric skillet for several reasons. First, the metal muffin pan fits inside it nicely, which allows me to create a makeshift double boiler to melt the wax in individual cups (more on this in the recipe section of this book). You can use a stovetop double boiler, but because beeswax is not water soluble, you will never be able to use that double boiler for any other purpose except making lotion bars.* You can also create a makeshift double boiler by heating an inch or two of water in a pan on the stove and melting your ingredients inside a glass mason jar which you set in the water.

*A NOTE ABOUT BEESWAX: BEESWAX IS NOT WATER SOLUBLE AND IS THEREFORE VERY DIFFICULT TO REMOVE FROM COOKWARE. TO MAKE LOTION BARS, WE DO *NOT* SUGGEST THAT YOU USE A TRADITIONAL DOUBLE BOILER, AS YOU WILL LIKELY NEVER BE ABLE TO GET THE WAX RESIDUE OUT OF THE PAN AGAIN. INSTEAD, CHOOSE A GLASS MASON JAR THAT YOU CAN DEDICATE TO THIS PURPOSE AND USE OVER AND OVER. WHATEVER TOOL YOU USE TO STIR THE MELTED LOTION INGREDIENTS WILL ALSO NEED TO BE DEDICATED TO THIS PURPOSE.

- **1 kitchen scale that will measure grams.** I measure each of the ingredients per bar for better accuracy and quality. To do this, I use an Ozeri® Pro Digital Kitchen Food Scale with a capacity of 1 gram to 12 pounds because this scale is capable of measuring quarter ounces. Measuring by weight makes your finished product more consistent.

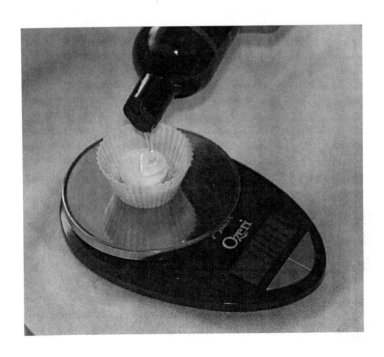

BASIC RECIPES

BASIC HARD LOTION BARS: SIMPLE METHOD

If you are making hard lotion bars for your own home use or to give as gifts to friends and family, the simple method will work best for you. The simple recipe may be scaled up, meaning you can double it, triple it, or make batches as large as you need.

- 1 ounce beeswax
- 1 ounce seed or nut butter
- 2 ounces oil

 STEP 1: Bring 2 inches of water to a gentle boil. Put ingredients in a glass mason jar and place the mason jar in the pan of boiling water. Stir the ingredients occasionally.

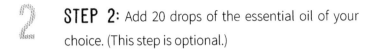

STEP 2: Add 20 drops of the essential oil of your choice. (This step is optional.)

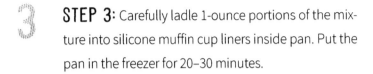

STEP 3: Carefully ladle 1-ounce portions of the mixture into silicone muffin cup liners inside pan. Put the pan in the freezer for 20–30 minutes.

STEP 4: When lotion bars are hardened, wrap them individually in cupcake wrappers and seal with a sticker if desired. Individual bars may be stored in 2.5-inch round tins.

Makes four 1-ounce bars.

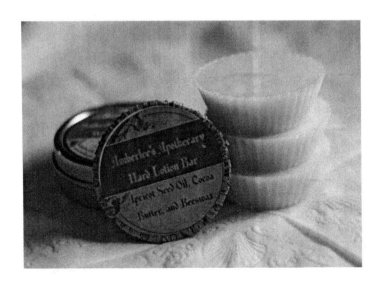

BASIC HARD LOTION BARS: COMMERCIALLY ACCURATE METHOD

If you are making lotion bars to sell, you will need to be more accurate in how you mix and weigh ingredients if you want to make sure each bar is of the highest quality. This is my recipe for making bars to sell. In this recipe, I measure the ingredients for each individual bar instead of measuring ingredients for a whole batch. This has several advantages. First, each bar ends up with the correct weight. Second, each bar ends up with the correct blend of ingredients. Third, there is no need to attempt to pour or measure melted oils and wax. (Accurately measuring the melted mixture can be difficult.) There is also less waste because you are not trying to pour hot liquid, a difficult task when you are trying to get an exact weight.

- 1/4 ounce beeswax
- 1/4 ounce seed or nut butter
- 1/2 ounce oil

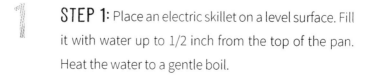

STEP 1: Place an electric skillet on a level surface. Fill it with water up to 1/2 inch from the top of the pan. Heat the water to a gentle boil.

STEP 2: Use 2 square wooden dowels across the top of the skillet to hang the metal muffin pan with silicone liners in the water. This ensures that the bottom of the pan is in the water but that the pan is high enough that boiling water doesn't splash into the molds, which would ruin your lotion bars.

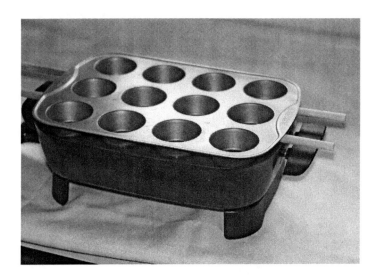

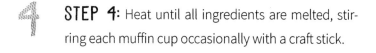

STEP 3: Measure out ingredients and place them in each individual muffin cup liner. You will put 1/4 ounce of pelleted beeswax into each of the 12 individual muffin cups followed by 1/4 ounce of seed or nut butter and 1/2 ounce of oil. Note that each muffin cup liner will hold more than an ounce, so they will not be full.

STEP 4: Heat until all ingredients are melted, stirring each muffin cup occasionally with a craft stick.

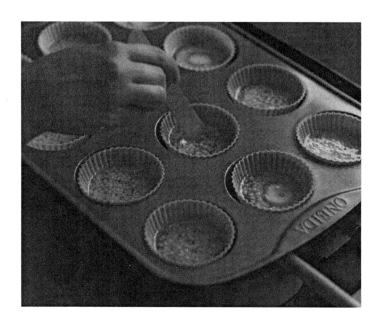

STEP 5: Add drops of the essential oil of your choice.* (This step is optional.)

*PEPPERMINT AND LAVENDER HAVE A STRONGER SMELL, AND THESE NEED 3 DROPS PER MUFFIN CUP. LEMON AND GRAPEFRUIT ESSENTIAL OILS HAVE A WEAKER SMELL, AND YOU WILL NEED 5 DROPS IF YOU ARE USING ONE OF THESE. WITH EXPERIENCE, YOU WILL BE ABLE TO DETERMINE WHETHER OTHER OILS HAVE A STRONG OR WEAK SMELL, AND THIS WILL DE-TERMINE HOW MUCH OIL IS NEEDED PER BAR.

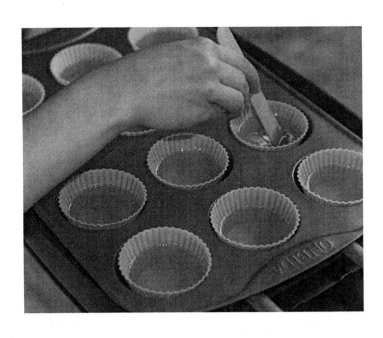

STEP 6: Turn off the skillet and carefully transfer the muffin pan to the fridge or freezer for 20 minutes.* The mixture may be left to harden at room temperature, but hardening at room temperature may cause the beeswax to separate. If you allow the bars to harden in the fridge or freezer, the beeswax will not separate.

*DO NOT SPILL THE HOT MIXTURE ON SKIN OR SEVERE BURNS MAY RESULT. IF YOU ARE BURNED, CALL FOR EMERGENCY HELP.

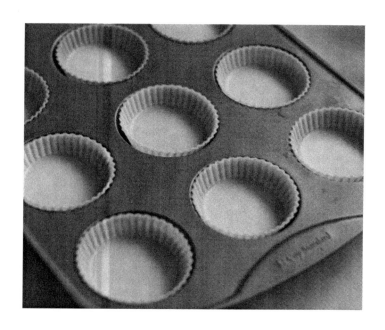

STEP 7: Once the lotion bars have completely cooked and hardened, package and label them.

TIP: I WRAP EACH BAR IN A PLAIN WHITE CUPCAKE WRAPPER AND THEN TURN IT OVER AND WRAP IT AGAIN IN A COLORFUL DESIGNER CUPCAKE WRAPPER. I USE THIS DOUBLE-WRAPPING METHOD BECAUSE THE WRAPPERS ARE NOT QUITE LARGE ENOUGH TO COVER THE WHOLE BAR IF I USE JUST ONE WRAPPER. I SEAL THE OUTER WRAPPER IN THE CENTER WITH AN AMBERLEE'S APOTHECARY LABEL, WHICH INCLUDES MY CONTACT INFORMATION FOR REORDERING.

Makes twelve 1-ounce bars.

RECIPE VARIATIONS

THE SIMPLE WHOLE-BODY BAR

This is the bar I use daily. This is good for full-body moisturizing and is compatible with all skin types.

- 2 ounces avocado oil
- 1 ounce cocoa butter
- 1 ounce beeswax

To make this bar, follow the basic lotion bar simple recipe. *Makes four 1-ounce bars or one 4-ounce bar.*

THE AFTER-SUN BAR

After spending all day in the sun, this is the bar to turn to. It contains rosehip oil, which helps heal sun-damaged skin.

- 0.2 ounces rosehip oil
- 1.8 ounces apricot kernel oil
- 1 ounce shea butter
- 1 ounce beeswax

To make this bar, follow the basic lotion bar simple recipe. After all ingredients are melted, add 20 drops of lavender essential oil, or add 5 drops to each individual bar after pouring. *Makes four 1-ounce bars or one 4-ounce bar.*

JUST FOR HEELS (OR HEALING) BAR

This bar is formulated especially for cracked and calloused skin, making it perfect for the heels of the feet or rough hands.

- 1.8 ounces avocado oil
- 1 ounce shea butter
- 1 ounce beeswax
- 0.1 ounces tamanu oil

To make this bar, follow the basic lotion bar simple recipe. After everything is melted, add 0.1 ounces evening primrose oil. Apply to feet immediately after washing them. *Makes four 1-ounce bars or one 4-ounce bar.*

HARD LOTION BAR STORAGE: ANY COVERED CONTAINER CAN BE USED TO STORE HARD LOTION BARS. I USE 2.5-INCH ROUND TINS, WHICH ARE INEXPENSIVE AND AVAILABLE ONLINE. WHEN I SELL LOTION BARS, I SELL THE TINS SEPARATELY OR GIVE AWAY ONE FREE TIN WHEN SELLING A SET OF THREE BARS. THE TINS MAKE IT EASY TO KEEP DUST OFF THE BARS, MAKE THE BARS EASY TO CARRY IN A PURSE, AND ARE PERFECT FOR TRAVEL.

STARTING A LOTION BAR BUSINESS

Starting my lotion bar business was accidental. Initially I was giving the bars away as gifts for Christmas and birthdays; I had not thought of selling them. I was actually trying to come up with a good Christmas stocking-stuffer that I thought people would actually use. When the recipients began asking for more bars, I started selling them to family members.

I regularly go to our farmers' market, and I thought I wanted to try to sell something because it looked fun. The rule at our local farmers' market is that what you sell has to be a handmade product, so lotion bars fit the requirements perfectly.

TIPS FOR SUCCESS AT THE FARMERS' MARKET

After several profitable seasons of selling at the farmers' market, I have some tips for success.

- Location at the market is important. Make sure there is good foot traffic near your table.

- Don't expect people to come up to you and ask what you are selling. You have to interact with the people passing by. I give away free samples of my lotion bars. When I offer samples, customers are usually grateful and curious about my product, giving me a chance to explain the homemade bars. This type of interaction will increase your chance of making a sale.

- Be careful. Sometimes when I give away free samples, over-eager customers eat them before I can finish explaining what they are. If I slowly begin, "Would you like a free sample . . . ?" they will have popped it in their mouth before I can finish my sentence. I have learned to quickly say, "Would you like a free lotion sample?"

PRICING

When I first started selling lotion bars, I asked friends and family if they would be willing to pay $5 per bar. When they agreed, I then looked on Etsy.com to research comparable prices for 1-ounce bars. I discovered that $5 is a standard market price and I set my price at $5 per bar. I quickly discovered, however, that people are likely to spend more if they have an incentive to purchase more than one bar at a time. To create this incentive, I offer a set of three bars for the price of two bars ($10 at this writing), and I include a metal storage tin as a free gift. To create further incentives, I offer a set of five bars for the price of three bars ($15 at this writing) with a free tin and a set of ten bars for the price of five bars ($25) with three free storage tins.

TIP: SETTING PRICES IN EVEN $5 INCREMENTS MAKES IT MUCH EASIER TO MAKE CHANGE AT THE MARKET.

PROFIT

To make a profit, you must take into consideration all of your expenses. Consider pricing carefully. Start by making a full list of your expenses.

- **Ingredients.** At this writing, it costs $1 for the ingredients to make a single 1-ounce lotion bar.
- **Storefront costs.** I pay $12 per week for my booth at the farmers market and a one-time yearly application fee of $25. I also must pay a percentage and listing fee when selling on Etsy.com.
- **Shipping and travel.** I have to pay for gas to get to and from the market and when shopping locally for supplies. I have to pay shipping if I order online.
- **Equipment.** I have to cover the cost of the equipment I use and any future replacements or upgrades. This includes the electric skillet, the muffin pan, the craft sticks, and the silicone liners.
- **Labels.** Buying labels in bulk from labelsonline.com usually results in the best price per label that I have been able to find (1,000 labels for about $20 at this writing). I also have to use a home color printer and ink cartridges to print my label sheets. Taking all this into consideration, my cost per label is about 10 cents. I designed my label using free online label design software from Vistaprint.com, and I have purchased labels from the site as well.
- **Packaging.** I package each bar in two cupcake wrappers. I pay $2 for 75 wrappers at the craft store. I use a white wrapper and a colored designer wrapper, and the price is the same for both.

- **Production time.** I have to be able to pay myself for the time it takes me to produce the bars.
- **Sales time.** I have to be able to pay myself for the time it takes me to sell the bars.
- **Investing in the business.** It is important to use part of the proceeds from your business to invest in growing the business. Here are some examples of how I have invested in my business:

  - I will soon use part of the profits from my business to purchase a higher-quality color printer for creating my product labels at home. The printer I use now costs about $90 but is slow and doesn't have high-end printing quality. I am investing in a new printer so that I can print labels faster and have higher printing resolution.
  - I have used part of the business income to experiment with new oils and essential oils for fragrances.
  - Looking to expand my product line, I have purchased what is necessary to begin selling homemade lip balm. I may also expand to offer other product lines or kits for making products at home.

EXPANDING YOUR BUSINESS

Becoming a profitable small business—very small, in my case—does not happen overnight. My immediate goal in joining the farmers' market was to make more money than it cost to rent the booth space, and I have always done that. I have never made less than the cost of the booth space. The farmers' market that I attend lasts four hours and is held weekly in Logan, Utah, over the course of four months, which is our summer season.

On my least profitable day ever, I took in just $30. This was on a day late in the season when the weather was cooler and the market—and the number of customers—was dwindling. On my best day ever, I took in $127. When considering whether this signifies a success or a failure, I have to consider my goals. If this were my full-time business, I would have to travel to sell at multiple farmers' markets, build up an online store, and foster a list of returning customers. I would also need to expand my product line. Because I have a full-time job as a chemist, I don't have to rely solely on the income from my small business—but this doesn't mean that I should run my business at a loss. It just means that I have the luxury of being able to grow my accidental business slowly, creating a base of returning customers while I consider new products.

Meanwhile, I have been paid for giving demonstrations on how to make lotion bars, and it was one of those demonstrations that led to writing this book. You never know where starting a small business might lead.

FREE OFFER: TO GET A FREE SAMPLE OF AMBERLEE'S ALL-NATURAL HARD LOTION, GO TO SEEDRENAISSANCE. COM, AND CLICK ON "FREE OFFERS."

FREQUENTLY ASKED QUESTIONS AND TROUBLESHOOTING

QUESTION: How do I use the lotion bar?

ANSWER: Rub the bar once or twice over the desired skin area; that is sufficient to melt a thin layer of the lotion. Then massage in the lotion.

QUESTION: I don't like any of the oils you listed for making hard lotion. Can I use one that I already know my skin will like?

ANSWER: Yes, any oil will do. A note about grapeseed oil: it is not very heat stable. If you use it in the hard lotion recipe, wait until all of the butter and wax are melted then add the grapeseed oil, stir, and remove mixture from heat.

QUESTION: Will I experience the medicinal properties of the essential oil I've added to the hard lotion?

ANSWER: Maybe. It depends on how much you add. I would recommend applying the essential oils directly to the skin after you have put on the hard lotion.

QUESTION: My beeswax is taking forever to melt; I don't like grating beeswax; beeswax is ruining my knives. What can I do?

ANSWER: Get beeswax pellets or beads instead, which are easy to melt and weigh out.

QUESTION: How long will my hard lotion bar last?

ANSWER: Hard lotion is shelf stable and won't need refrigeration because there is no water. Most of the bar ingredients have about a one-year shelf life. As long as you keep your hard lotion bar away from moisture and minimize its exposure to air, it will last a year. I make my hard lotion in batches to last a few months and keep the bars between sheets of parchment paper. The hard lotion bars I use for just my hands usually take about three months to be completely used up. I use a little over an ounce per week for whole body moisturizing, but I have a petite body, so other people might use more.

QUESTION: Where can I buy all of these ingredients?

ANSWER: If you don't yet know what oils and butters you are going to use, I would suggest getting small quantities from your local health food store to experiment with so you're not stuck with a whole gallon of oil you can't use. If you know what you are going to use, buy online in bulk. There are many bulk suppliers that sell high-quality ingredients, but keep in mind that you don't want to buy too much that will expire before you are able to use it.

QUESTION: Do the bars make good gifts?

ANSWER: Yes. Everyone who has received a bar from me has commented on how nice the bars are.

QUESTION: Can I use beeswax that I've processed myself?

ANSWER: Yes, and you will retain most of the beeswax's antimicrobial properties along with all the healthful properties of the small amounts of honey that will be left in the wax. Your hard lotion may also have a light honey smell to it.

QUESTION: Water accidently got into my hard lotion bar while I was making it; is it still good to use?

ANSWER: That depends on how much water, and if it was emulsified into the hard lotion. If you can see water droplets on the bottom of your container, the end product will be okay; the lotion bar will harden around the droplets, and you can wipe them up after the hard lotion is solid. If you spilled a lot of water and your hard lotion starts to froth, it has become emulsified with the water. Chances are that water wasn't distilled or sterile and probably has bacteria in it, even though it has been boiled. I personally wouldn't risk it and would throw it away.

QUESTION: After I used my hard lotion bar all up, there were little hard parts that wouldn't melt on my skin.

ANSWER: That is beeswax. It means that you didn't stir your ingredients well enough; stir better next time.

QUESTION: Someone has accidentally ingested my hard lotion bar; is that bad?

ANSWER: All of the ingredients I have listed are also used in food preparation and are completely edible as long as they are cold pressed or expeller pressed.

QUESTION: I have developed a skin rash from my hard lotion.

ANSWER: Try testing the ingredients individually on your skin first to make sure that you won't have a reaction. Make sure you are getting high-quality ingredients. Try a different oil or butter.

QUESTION: Is this hard lotion recipe just a salve?

ANSWER: No, salves are only a mixture of oil and beeswax. They are also soft at room temperature; my hard lotion is a completely solid at room temperature.

QUESTION: Can I add more than one oil or butter to my hard lotion?

ANSWER: Yes, you may do any combination of oils and butters for your hard lotion; just be sure that the oil portion is two parts and that the butter portion is one part to maintain correct consistency.

QUESTION: Will hard lotion fix all of my skin problems?

ANSWER: No, healthy skin starts from the inside out. Your skin is the first exit for anything toxic in your diet. If your body can't push the toxins out through the skin, the toxins will move on to the liver and kidneys. Eat clean foods and drink clean water. It can take up to six months for your skin to heal completely, so be patient.

QUESTION: Can I just use a natural oil to moisturize my skin instead of a lotion bar?

ANSWER: Some people moisturize with straight oil, and it works for them, but when I tried that, I always felt like something was missing. I never felt like the oil protected my skin, and the oil was missing the moisturizing properties of lotion. When I used straight oil, a little while later I would have to put more on. It never really gave my skin moisture. I do, however, use just oil on my face since the hard lotion can feel heavy. I use jojoba oil on my face because it is recommended for acne-prone skin and because it has a chemical makeup similar to sebum, the natural oils your body produces. I put it on in the morning after I wash my face.

DEfiniTiOnS

CAMPAIGN FOR SAFE COSMETICS: A coalition dedicated to protecting consumers from chemicals used in cosmetics that are linked with cancer, birth defects, and other health problems.

EMOLLIENT: A substance that softens and soothes skin.

EMULSIFIER: A substances that mixes oil with water.

ENVIRONMENTAL WORKING GROUP: An organization that researches and advocates against the use of toxic chemicals in food and care products.

ESSENTIAL OIL: The oil that is produced by a plant or flower when it is pressed or distilled. Essential oils can have medicinal properties.

HUMECTANT: A substance that pulls moisture from the air into skin.

LIPID: Another term for oil or fat.

MOISTURIZER: A substance that includes an oil, an emollient, and a humectant.

OXIDIZED: Describes the state of a substance after it reacts with oxygen, changing the substance's properties.

SUPPLY SOURCES

- Amazon.com: For small quantities and experimenting, NOW brands of oils and butters are well priced, but be sure to check extraction methods.
- BulkApothecary.com: A good source for large quantities of cold and expeller pressed oils.
- PaperMart.com: A good source for 2.5-inch metal storage tins.
- RoseMountainHerbs.com: A good source to order organic oils in bulk.
- SeedRenaissance.com: The place to buy Amberlee's Apothecary lotion bars online.
- SoapGoods.com: A good source for smaller quantities of non-organic but still cold- and expeller-pressed oils.

SOURCES

1. *Fooducate.com*. "What Is Expeller Pressed Oil and Why Does It Matter?" December 8, 2010. www.blog.Fooducate.com/2010/12/08/what-is-expeller-pressed-oil-and-why-does-it-matter/

2. Agency for Toxic Substances and Disease Registry. "Toxic Facts™ for Hexane." June 1999. Last updated May 6, 2014. www.ATSDR.cdc.gov/toxfaqs/tf.asp?id=392&tid=68

3. Blechman, Nicholas. "Extra Virgin Suicide." *The New York Times*. January 24, 2014. www.NYTimes.com/interactive/2014/01/24/opinion/food-chains-extra-virgin-suicide.html?_r=0

ABOUT THE AUTHORS

AMBERLEE RYNN is the founder and owner of Amberlee's Apothecary, where she manufacturers scented and unscented hard lotion bars, natural lip balms, and other products, in addition to teaching lotion-making classes. Her products are sold at SeedRenaissance.com, on Etsy.com, and at local farmers' markets. Amberlee has a bachelor's degree in chemistry from Utah Valley University and works as a full-time forensic chemist for the state of Utah.

ALEB WARNOCK is the popular author of *Forgotten Skills of Self-Sufficiency Used by the Mormon Pioneers*, *The Art of Baking with Natural Yeast*, *Backyard Winter Gardening For All Climates*, *More Forgotten Skills*, *Trouble's On The Menu*, and more. He is the owner of SeedRenaissance.com and blogs at CalebWarnock.blogspot.com, where you will find a link to join his email list to learn more about forgotten skills.

ABOUT FAMILIUS

VISIT OUR WEBSITE: www.familius.com

JOIN OUR FAMILY: There are lots of ways to connect with us! Subscribe to our newsletters at www.familius.com to receive uplifting daily inspiration, essays from our Pater Familius, a free ebook every month, and the first word on special discounts and Familius news.

GET BULK DISCOUNTS: If you feel a few friends and family might benefit from what you've read, let us know and we'll be happy to provide you with quantity discounts. Simply email us at specialorders@familius.com.

CONNECT:

www.facebook.com/paterfamilius
@familiustalk, @paterfamilius1
www.pinterest.com/familius

FAMILIUS

THE MOST IMPORTANT WORK YOU EVER DO WILL BE WITHIN THE WALLS OF YOUR OWN HOME.